# CHAIR YOGA FOR SENIORS OVER 60

## Enjoy a Peaceful Yoga Session without Leaving Your Seat

## Mark Jayce

COPYWRIGHT PAGE

Copyright © 2023 by [Mark Jayce]

TABLE OF CONTENTS

# INTRODUCTION

Embracing her love for promoting happiness and health among seniors over 60, Funke, a lively woman with a warm smile, pursued her goal. She knew how vital it was to stay active and maintain a happy view on life because she had personally witnessed the difficulties of old age via her own grandparents.

A group of excited seniors looked forward to Funke's straightforward chair yoga classes at the neighborhood community center every morning when she showed up. As Funke led them through easy stretches and tranquil breathing exercises, the light, sunny room erupted in laughter and companionship.

The elders gained newfound flexibility and strength with each day that went by. They loved the sense of accomplishment they got from performing movements they had assumed were no longer possible as they became older. The meetings were made enjoyable by Funke's patience and compassion, and each person's life was changed for the better by her sincere concern for them.

The elders' emotional and physical health got better throughout the course of the weeks. They developed solid relationships with one another, offering one other the friendship and support that was required. A welcome break from their boring days, the chair yoga practice developed into a beloved component of their routines.

The work Funke did gave her satisfaction, too. Her heart was filled with excitement as she saw the changes in her kids and realized how she had contributed to their improvement. She was thankful for the chance to influence the people she came in contact with.

Funke noticed a new face among the seniors one day when the group of students assembled for their regular lesson. After losing her longtime companion, a lady by the name of Margaret had recently moved there in search of comfort. With her eyes heavy with sorrow, Margaret exuded apprehension.

Funke came over to Margaret and gave her a warm hug, assuring her that she was at a place that was secure and friendly. Funke gave Margaret special attention during the entire session, gently encouraging her as she moved through the poses. A glimmer of optimism appeared in Margaret's eyes as her guarded posture gradually relaxed.

Margaret began showing up frequently in the ensuing weeks as she found solace in the encouraging group that Funke had created. Margaret was able to heal physically and mentally thanks to the chair yoga sessions. She gained newfound resilience and a feeling of purpose.

As chair yoga gained popularity among the seniors, more people from nearby areas started to attend. Funke's little project grew into a thriving program that gave many seniors happiness, companionship, and life.

Many others were inspired by Funke's experience teaching chair yoga to elders over 60. It showed the power of an uncomplicated notion motivated by compassion and how it might change lives and build a close-knit society woven together by the threads of wellbeing, happiness, and togetherness.

# CHAPTER 1

## *MEANING OF YOGA*

India is the country where yoga, an age-old holistic discipline, first appeared. The goal of this approach is to attain harmony and balance in a person's life by including all facets of their physical, mental, and spiritual well-being. The word "yoga" derives from the Sanskrit root "yuj," which means to join or combine. It refers to the joining of the personal self with the greater, universal self in this context.

Yoga is made up of a variety of methods and exercises that can be customized to meet the demands of varied people. In the West, the physical practice of yoga, or "asana," which entails adopting various positions and postures to enhance the body's flexibility, strength, and balance, is the most well-known and well-liked part of the discipline.

But yoga incorporates other crucial elements that go beyond just physical exercise:

Exercises for controlling and regulating the breath, which is thought to be the source of life force or "prana," are called pranayama.

Methods to acquire mental clarity, focus, and relaxation through the practice of meditation. Yoga incorporates meditation as a crucial component since it helps people develop self-awareness and mindfulness.

Sacred words or sounds are said aloud as a mantra to improve focus and spiritual ties.

A practitioner's interactions with oneself, others, and their environment are governed by the yamas and niyamas, or ethical rules and principles.

Dhyana: Constant contemplation and meditation to advance one's spiritual practice.

The highest level of self-realization, referred to as samadhi, is one in which the practitioner feels profoundly connected to and at one with the universe.

Although yoga is not associated with any particular religion, it is frequently linked to the spiritual and intellectual teachings of old Indian faiths like Hinduism and Buddhism. Nowadays, many people turn to yoga as a way to improve their entire quality of life, reduce stress, improve their physical health, and enhance their mental well-being. All across the world, individuals of different ages and religions engage in it.

# CHAPTER 2

## *MEANING OF CHAIR YOGA AND ITS FORMS*

Originating in ancient India thousands of years ago, yoga is a comprehensive system of mental, physical, and spiritual exercises. One of the core components of practicing yoga is performing yoga poses, sometimes referred to as asanas. They entail a series of postures and motions that are meant to strengthen, stretch, balance, and sharpen the mind.

With an emphasis on correct alignment and breath awareness, yoga activities are often performed slowly and deliberately. Yoga emphasizes the connection between the breath and each movement, and practitioners are encouraged to do so in order to develop a sense of harmony and flow.

Yoga exercises come in a wide variety with varying goals and advantages. The following are a few well-liked yoga styles:

Hatha Yoga is a core style of yoga that is gentle and emphasizes breathing control and fundamental poses.

**Vinyasa** Yoga is a dynamic, flowing form of yoga where the breath and the movements are coordinated.

**Ashtanga Yoga:** A more strenuous and organized type of yoga that adheres to a predetermined order of poses.

**Bikram Yoga:** Also referred to as "hot yoga," it entails a predetermined sequence of 26 postures and two breathing exercises that are performed in a heated environment.

Precision and alignment are stressed in Iyengar yoga, which frequently uses straps and blocks as props to help practitioners hold poses.

**Kundalini Yoga:** Involves chanting, breathwork, and dynamic movements as it focuses on reawakening the energy at the base of the spine.

A slow-moving form of yoga that encourages flexibility and relaxation by holding positions for a long time is known as yin yoga.

The physical and mental health of oneself are both enhanced by yoga workouts. Regular practice helps to create inner serenity and balance while reducing stress and enhancing attention and concentration.

When practicing yoga, especially if you are a beginner, it is imperative to follow the instructions of a certified instructor to make sure you are doing the poses safely and correctly. Before beginning a new yoga practice, like with any physical exercise, it's a good idea to speak with a healthcare provider, especially if you have any underlying medical issues or injuries.

# CHAPTER 3

## *40 SIMPLE CHAIR YOGA FOR SENIORS OVER 60*

Seniors over 60 can benefit greatly from chair yoga, which they can do while relaxing in a chair and increasing their strength, flexibility, and general health. The following 40 easy chair yoga poses are suitable for seniors and quick to perform:

1.Sit tall and place your feet flat on the floor in the seated mountain pose while placing your hands on your thighs. Taking a deep breath, extend your spine.

2. From a seated position, reach for your toes or shins with your extended arms and slowly bend at the hips.

3. Twist while seated by placing one hand on the knee across from the other and slowly rotating the torso to the side. On the other side, repeat.

**4. Cat-Cow position while seated:** Take a deep breath, arch your back, and look upward. In the "Cat Pose," exhale, round the back, and tuck the chin.

5. Roll your shoulders in a smooth circular motion, first moving them forward, then moving them back.

6. Stretching the neck involves gently rolling it in a half-circle while tilting the head slowly to one side, then the other.

7. Stretch one arm overhead while seated in a warrior position. Lean to the side you are leaning toward. On the other side, repeat.

8. Lifting one foot off the ground, turn the ankle in a circle. Switch feet after reiterating in the reverse direction.

9. To open the chest and shoulders while seated, clasp your hands behind your back and extend your arms straight.

10. Stretching the wrists involves extending one arm in front of you with the palm facing down and bending the fingers slightly toward the floor.

11. Bring your feet's soles together while seated, and grasp your ankles while extending your knees out to the sides. Knees should be lightly raised and lowered.

12. Stretch one leg out straight and flex the foot while seated to perform leg lifts. A few inches off the ground, raise the leg, then hold it there before lowering it. On the other side, repeat.

13. With one leg straight back and the toes flat on the floor, perform a high lunge while seated. To extend the front of the hip, lean slightly forward. On the other side, repeat.

14. When sitting, lean to the side while raising one arm overhead. This will give you a mild stretch. On the other side, repeat.

15. From the butterfly posture, slowly lean forward from the hips to experience a stretch in the lower back and inner thighs.

16. Crossing one leg over the knee of the other while seated allows you to do a simple side-to-side twist. On the other side, repeat.

17. Cross one ankle over the other knee while in a seated position for Figure 4 Stretch. Then, gently press the lifted knee toward the floor. On the other side, repeat.

18. Stretching the ankle across the knee while seated involves gradually pressing the lifted knee toward the floor while crossing the other ankle over it.

19. Hands on the chair's seat, back arched, chest lifted, and eyes directed forward in the seated cobra position.

20. Relaxing when seated requires that you close your eyes, sit comfortably, take long breaths, and concentrate on letting your body relax.

21. Take a seat in the mountain pose, placing your hands on your knees and sitting tall with your feet flat on the floor. Breathe deeply.

22. When seated, inhale, raise your arms, exhale, and bend forward at the hips, reaching for your feet.

23. **Twist when seated:** With your left hand on the outside of your left knee, gently twist to the left while glancing over your left shoulder. On the other side, repeat.

24. **Neck stretch:** Drop your right ear toward your right shoulder, then maintain the position for a few seconds. On the other side, repeat.

25. Rolling your shoulders back and forth will help you relieve stress.

26. **Ankle and Wrist Circles**: To increase joint mobility, rotate your ankles and wrists both clockwise and counterclockwise.

27. **Squatting Cat-Cow:** Take a deep breath, arch your back, and look upward (Cow). Pull your chin in and inhale while doing these three things (Cat).

28. Cross your right leg over your left and slowly rotate your torso to the right while seated in a spinal twist position. On the other side, repeat.

29. **Leg lifts while seated**: Raise one leg at a time and hold it straight out in front of you for a few seconds.

30. One knee should be hugged to the chest while you are seated. Repeat the process with the other knee.

31. Crossing the right ankle over the left knee in the ankle-to-knee position will give you a stretch in your hip. Gently press down on the right knee. On the other side, repeat.

32. Cross your right ankle over your left knee in the pigeon pose while sitting upright. You can feel a stretch in your hip by gently pushing your right knee away from you. On the other side, repeat.

33. In a straight-backed position, stretch your hamstrings by extending one leg straight out and reaching for your toes.

34. To expand your shoulders and lift your chest while seated, clasp your hands behind your back and extend your arms.

35. Stretch up towards the ceiling while sitting tall and in the seated warrior pose.

36. In the seated Eagle Arms position, bring your palms together, cross your right arm over your left, and place them in front of you. Hold on while changing sides.

37. **Seated Sun Salutation:** Perform this modified variation of the Sun Salutation, which includes bending and twisting your arms.

38. **Child's Pose in a seated position:** Place your forehead on the chair while sitting back on your heels and spreading your arms out in front of you.

39. In a seated meditation position, close your eyes, pay attention to your breathing, and engage in a brief session of mindfulness.

40. Seated Relaxation: Spend a few minutes unwinding and reaping the rewards of your practice as you finish your chair yoga session.

In particular, if you have pre-existing medical concerns, it is crucial to speak with a healthcare provider before beginning any new fitness regimen. As you practice chair yoga, take time to enjoy yourself and adjust as necessary to maintain your comfort and safety.

# CHAPTER 4

# BENEFITS OF YOGA CHAIR FOR SENIORS OVER 60

Seniors over 60 who practice chair yoga can reap a number of advantages, making it a convenient and efficient form of exercise. Some of the main advantages are listed below:

**Improved Flexibility:** Seniors can increase their flexibility by doing chair yoga, which entails moderate stretches and motions. The range of motion in joints can be expanded with regular practice, reducing stiffness and facilitating daily tasks.

**Strengthening**: Chair yoga is a mild kind of exercise, yet it nevertheless works a variety of muscle groups, enhancing both strength and stability. The risk of falls and injuries can be decreased through muscular strengthening by improving posture and balance.

**Tension reduction**: Chair yoga involves breathing exercises and meditation methods that can assist seniors in controlling their tension and anxiety. A peaceful, relaxed state is encouraged by mindful breathing, which enhances mental health as a whole.

**Joint Health:** Chair yoga is a low-impact exercise that is kind to the joints and is a good choice for elderly people who suffer from arthritis or other joint-related conditions. Joint stiffness and soreness can be reduced with regular practice.

**Circulation Enhanced:** Chair yoga's gentle motions and stretches can enhance circulation. A healthier heart and reduced edema in the legs and feet can also be benefits of enhanced circulation.

**Enhanced Mind-Body Connection**: Chair yoga can promote a greater connection between the mind and the body through attentive movement and Breath awareness. Better self-consciousness and a feeling of body control can result from this elevated awareness.

**Interaction with Others**: Seniors who take chair yoga courses have the chance to socialize with others and get involved in the community. It can help people feel more a part of a community and less alone.

**Pain relief:** Through mild stretches and relaxation methods, chair yoga practice on a regular basis may help reduce chronic pain, such as lower back pain or muscle tension.

**Improved Sleep:** The relaxation techniques employed in chair yoga can aid seniors in getting a better night's sleep by encouraging relaxation and minimizing sleep interruptions brought on by tension or discomfort.

**Flexibility:** Chair yoga is simply adaptable to meet the demands and physical limitations of each person. It is a flexible and inclusive form of exercise since it is appropriate for senior citizens with various levels of mobility and fitness.

**Increased Energy**: Chair yoga practice might help you feel more refreshed and energized. Throughout the day, seniors may feel more vivacious and enthusiastic.

# CONCLUSION

Conclusion: For seniors over 60, chair yoga is a very useful and practical type of exercise. In order to promote general wellbeing and lower the chance of injuries, it is more crucial for people to maintain their flexibility, strength, and balance as they age. For seniors, regardless of their physical capabilities or limitations, chair yoga offers a pleasant and safe option for them to exercise regularly.

Assisting older persons in meeting their unique needs by using modified postures and gentle movements, chair yoga helps them increase their range of motion, muscle tone, and joint flexibility. Additionally, the practice of chair yoga gives elders a chance to improve their mental health by developing awareness, stress reduction, and relaxation.

One of chair yoga's main benefits is that everyone can take part in the exercise, regardless of their degree of fitness or mobility issues. This fosters a feeling of community and encourages older citizens to interact with one another. Being able to overcome loneliness and isolation, which are common problems for elderly people, makes this feature particularly crucial.

Additionally, chair yoga can be used as an adjunctive therapy for treating several age-related illnesses like osteoporosis, arthritis, and persistent pain. Those who are suffering with these diseases can maintain or enhance their physical health without putting undue stress on their bodies thanks to its soft nature, which makes it a safe and reliable solution.

Health care providers, senior centers, and community organizations are increasingly including chair yoga in their senior programs as more research demonstrates its advantages. The advantages chair yoga can provide for older folks' quality of life are becoming more recognized.

 Chair yoga offers seniors over 60 a comprehensive approach to wellbeing, boosting their mental, emotional, and physical well-being. Due to its adaptability and accessibility, it is the perfect form of exercise for older people, allowing them to live more active, meaningful lives that are enriched by their elder years. Chair yoga, with its plethora of advantages and worldwide popularity, is unquestionably a useful and empowering practice for seniors looking to enhance their general quality of life.

Dear seniors,

Thank you from the bottom of our hearts for joining us in our journey through "Quick and Simple Chair Yoga for seniors over 60." Your dedication to staying active and nurturing your well-being is truly inspiring.

As we flowed through gentle stretches and calming breaths together, we witnessed the power of chair yoga to unlock a newfound sense of vitality and inner peace. Your enthusiasm and openness to try new movements warmed our souls.

Remember, age is just a number, and through this practice, we've learned that our bodies and spirits are resilient and capable of incredible transformations. May this chair yoga journey continue to bring you joy, strength, and a renewed sense of connection with yourself.

Your participation has made this experience even more meaningful, and we are grateful to have shared this special time with you. Keep spreading the light of positivity and good health as you inspire those around you to embrace the beauty of chair yoga.

With heartfelt thanks,

[Mark Jayce]